Whöösh!

Katie Brööke

pinter
&
martin

Whoosh! A little book for birth companions

First published by Pinter & Martin Ltd 2015

© 2015 Katie Brooke

Katie Brooke has asserted her moral rights to be identified as the author of this work in accordance with the Copyright, Designs and Patents Act of 1988.

ISBN 978-1-78066-185-8

British Library Cataloguing-in-Publication Data
A catalogue record for this book is available from the British Library.

Quote from *Ina May's Guide to Childbirth* (Vermilion, 2008) reprinted by kind permission of Ina May Gaskin and from *Well Adjusted Babies* by kind permission of Dr Jennifer Barham-Floreani www.welladjustedbabies.com

Printed and bound in China by Everbest Printing Co. Ltd.

Pinter & Martin Ltd, 6 Effra Parade, London SW2 1PS

pinterandmartin.com

for Steven

A book for

. . . .

with love

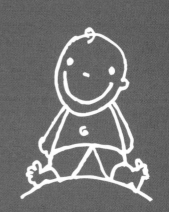

IF YOU'RE
READING THIS...

THEN

We're having a

BABY!

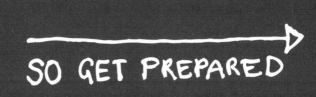

SO GET PREPARED

And
discover
unknown

ANIMAL
INSTINCTS!

SO: HERE ARE
SOME USEFUL
THINGS FOR YOU;
SOME STUFF TO
REMIND ME TO DO;
AND GENERALLY A
BOOK OF THINGS TO
DISTRACT
AND
AMUSE

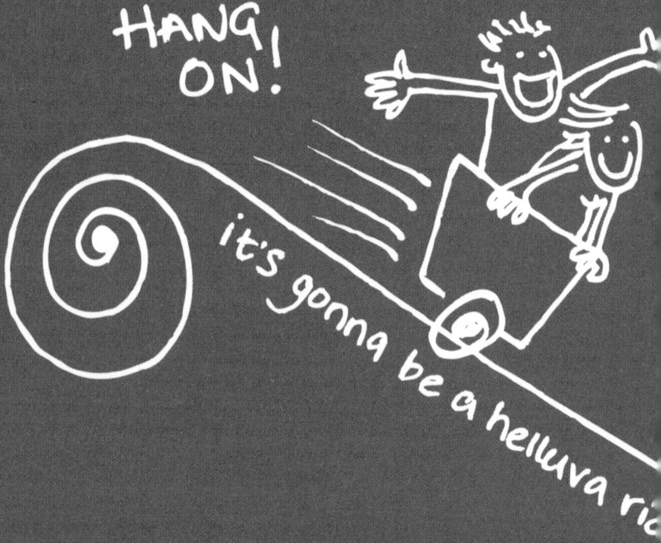

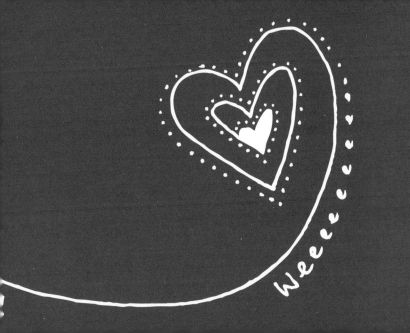

weeeeeee

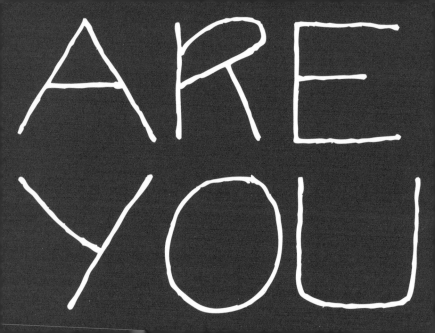

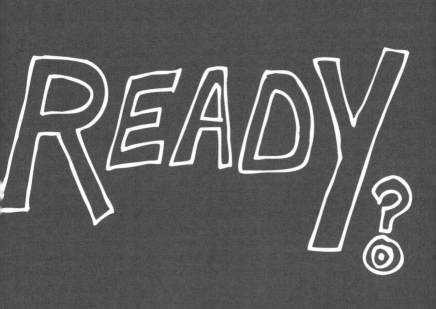

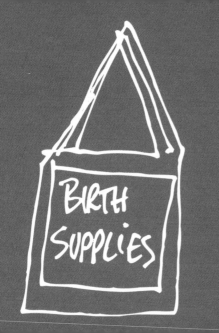

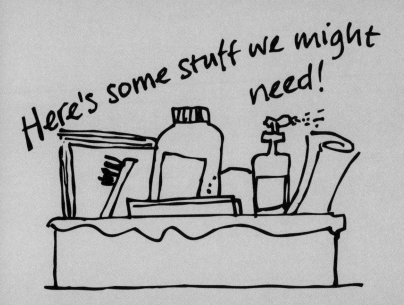

A jar of
Dead Nice Honey
for ENERGY!
∴∵∴∵∴∵∴∵∴

Mmmmmmmmmm.....

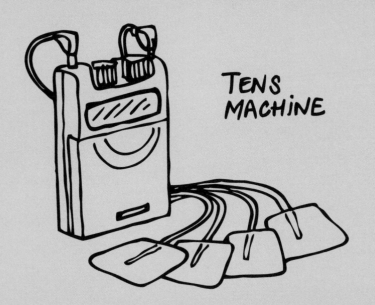

TENS MACHINE

LET'S LISTEN TO:

Snacks for me

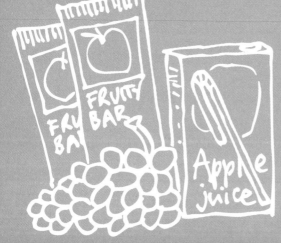
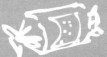

and for you!

ENERGY
FRUITFIZZ

CHOCBAR

Tennis Balls!

(what are these for?!)

..... MASSAGE !

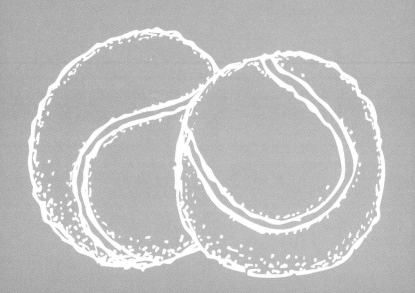

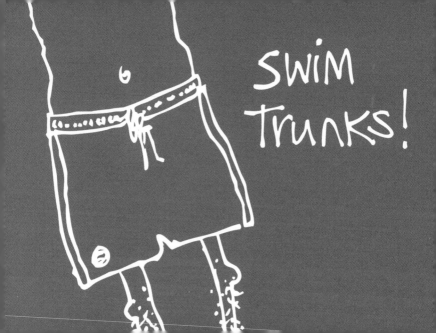

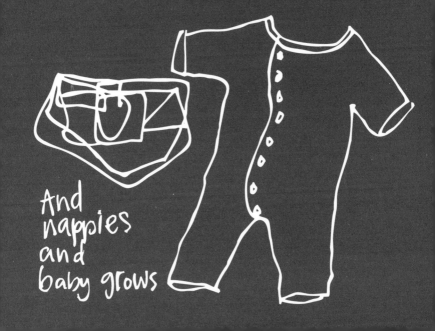

And
nappies
and
baby grows

THERE ARE ALSO 2 FLANNELS:

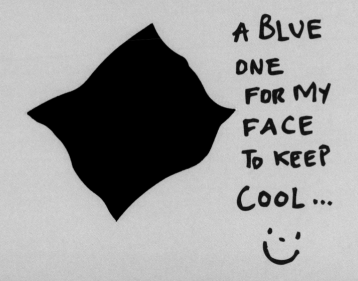

A BLUE
ONE
FOR MY
FACE
TO KEEP
COOL...

AND A
PINK
ONE
FOR A
HOT
PRESS
ON MY
PERINEUM

(fanny!)

and…

the rest
of it is bits
and bobs for
staying over
mostly....

....but

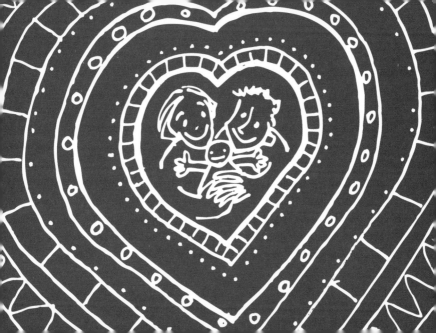

EXTRA BITS FOR YOU:

AND NOW FOR THE SCIENCE BIT →

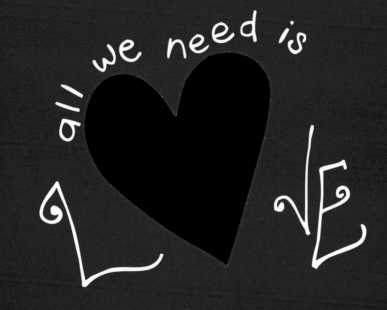

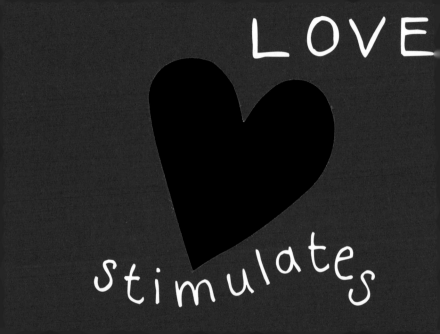

OXYTOCIN

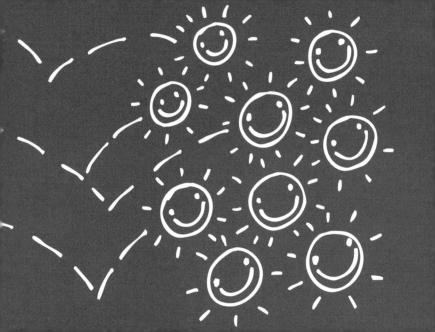

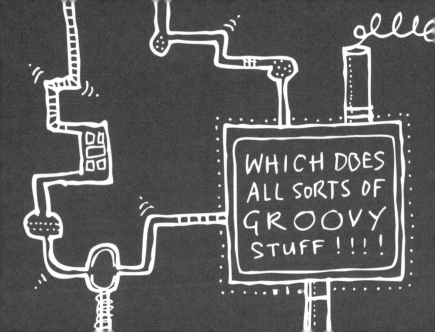

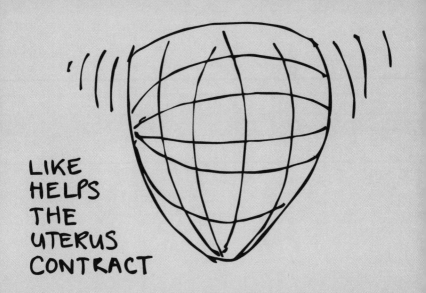

LIKE
HELPS
THE
UTERUS
CONTRACT

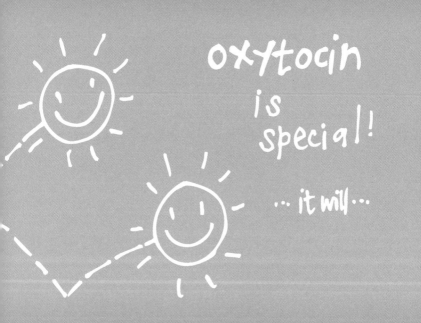

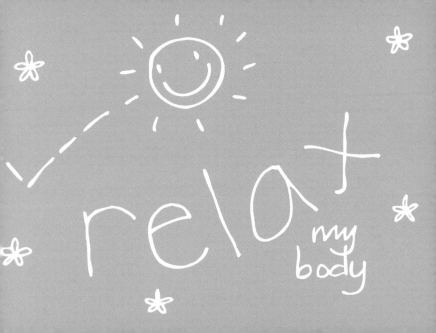

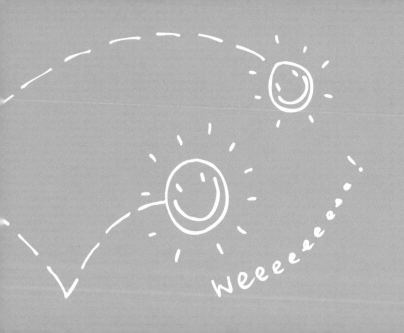

Weeeeeeee!

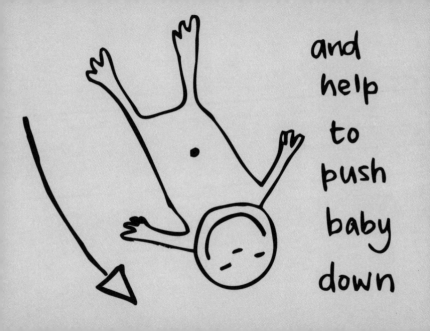

and
help
to
push
baby
down

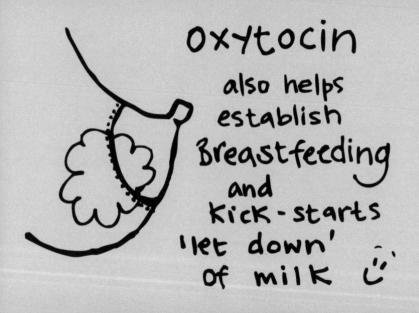

Whereas

ADRENALIN

IS <u>BAD NEWS</u> FOR LABOUR

ADRENALIN slows everything down and can even stop or reverse labour.

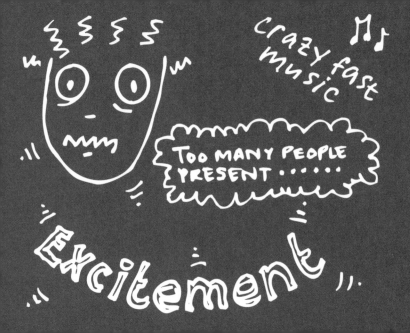

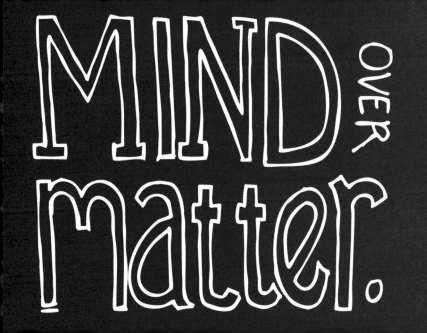

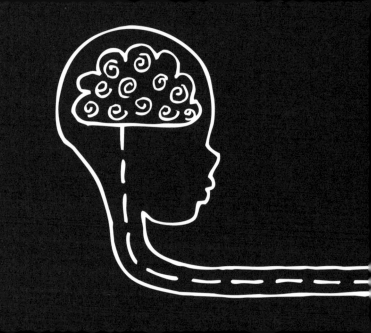

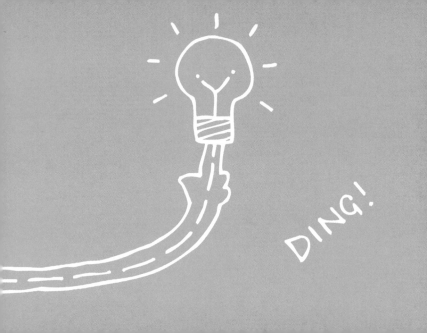

DING!

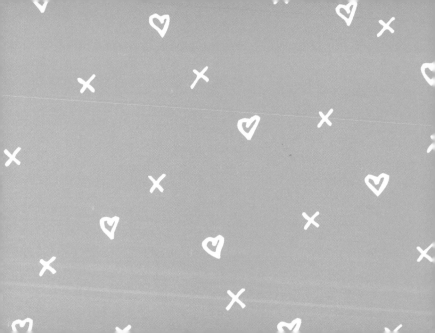

in which case...
let's give this brain
Some lovely nice things
to get it going...

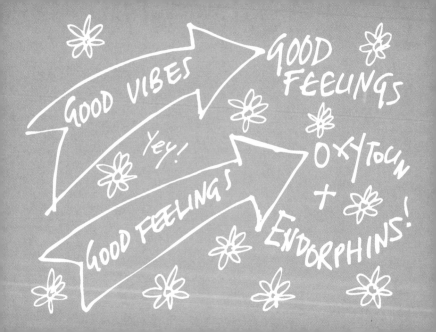

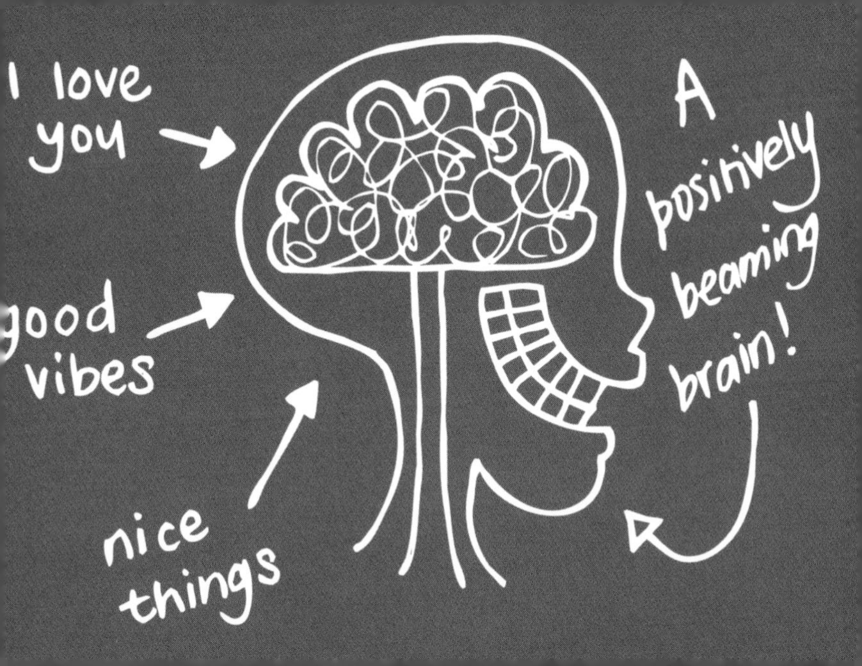
I love you
good vibes
nice things
A positively beaming brain!

and also...

dancing and laughing

feeling loved and supported

and above all...

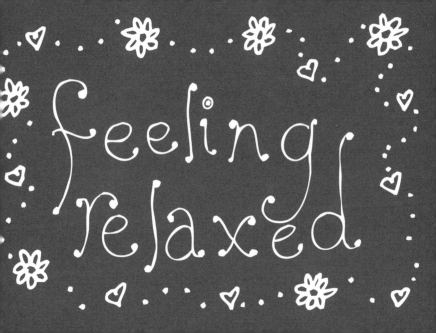

which is "really important"

Here we go!!!

♡♡♡ ♡♡♡♡ ♡♡ ♡♡♡♡ ♡♡♡♡♡♡♡ ♡♡

play some funky tunes MR DJ!

DANCE

Let's

Let's

Let's SING

LAUGH

Let's

Let's MOVE

Let's BE

TOGETHER

i06am!Here!Weeeee!

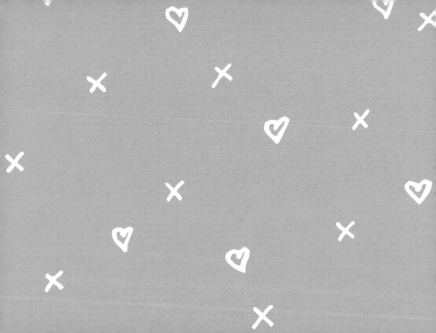

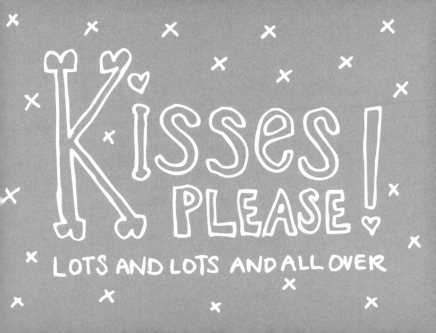

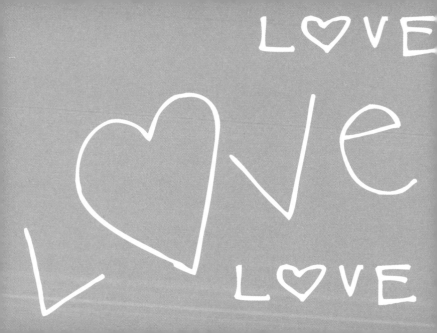

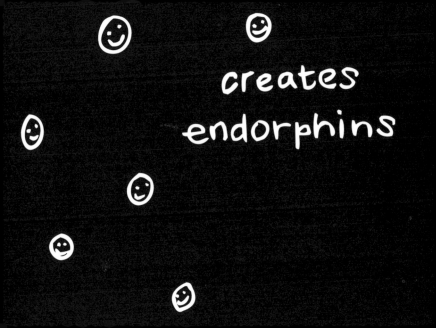

ENDORPHINS ARE NATURE'S OPIATES

Hurray for endorphins!

massage

Gets the endorphins going

... making me
feel all lovely and
Relaxed...

mmmmmmm....

massage #1

Gentle skin
surface strokes
with back of
your hands

(stimulates
receptors under
the skin
apparently!)

massage #2

Neck
and
shoulders
please!

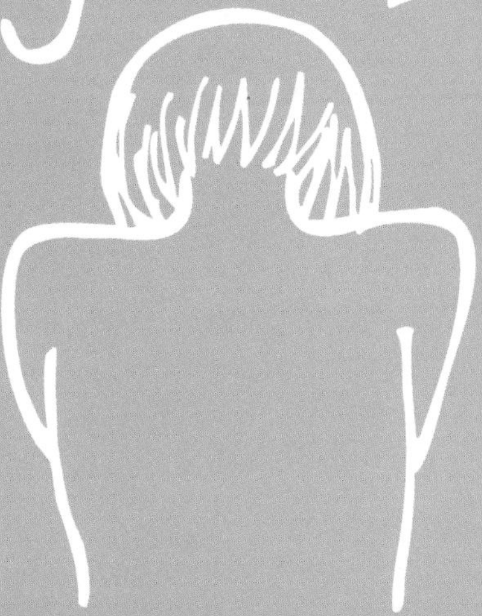

Oooh! Lovely!

massage # 3

The magic spot

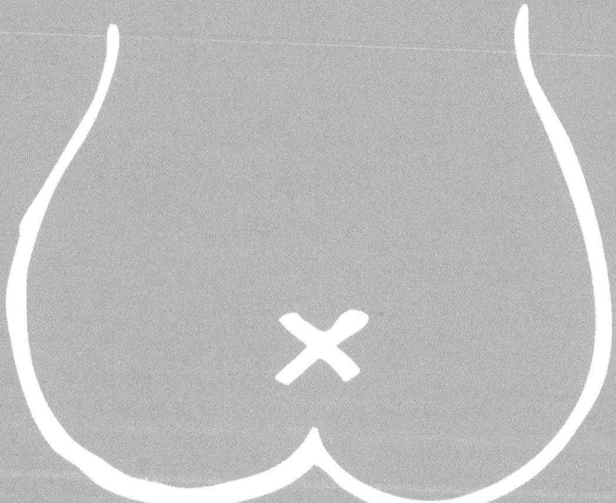

massage #4

the thigh shake!!

SERIOUSLY!
if I'm tense
grab those
thighs and
shake em!

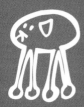

use the
funny
head
massage
thing

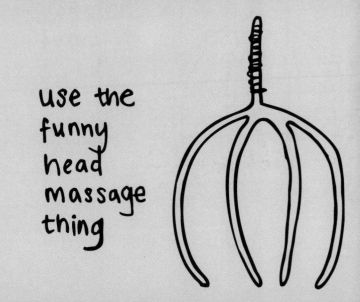

(I did wash them!)

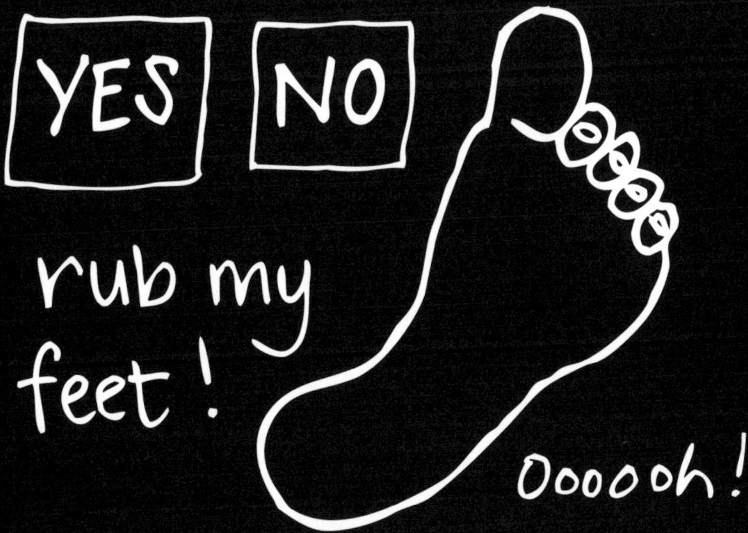
YES
NO
rub my feet!
Ooooh!

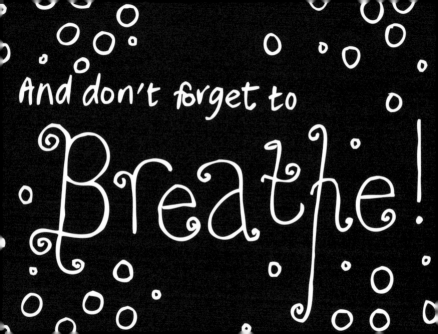

breathe

allow shoulders to drooooop...

Relax...

breathe out slowly...

relax

when it's happening...

...soft ...slow... quiet...

...long...quiet...slow...breaths...

Remind me to take a
deep breath
after each
Contraction...

O2

...Oxygen is important for baby too!

ENDORPHINS ACTUALLY BLOCK THE RECEPTION OF PAIN AND GIVE US A FEELING OF PLEASURE

Things to help PAIN.

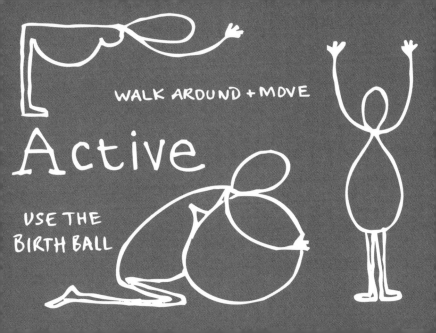

WALK AROUND + MOVE

Active

USE THE
BIRTH BALL

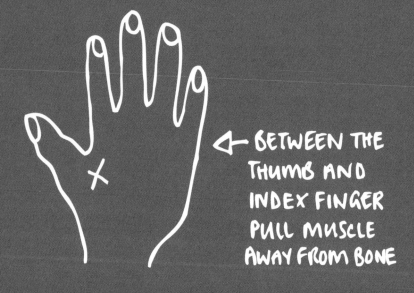

BETWEEN THE THUMB AND INDEX FINGER PULL MUSCLE AWAY FROM BONE

ACUPRESSURE POINTS

(easy and effective!)

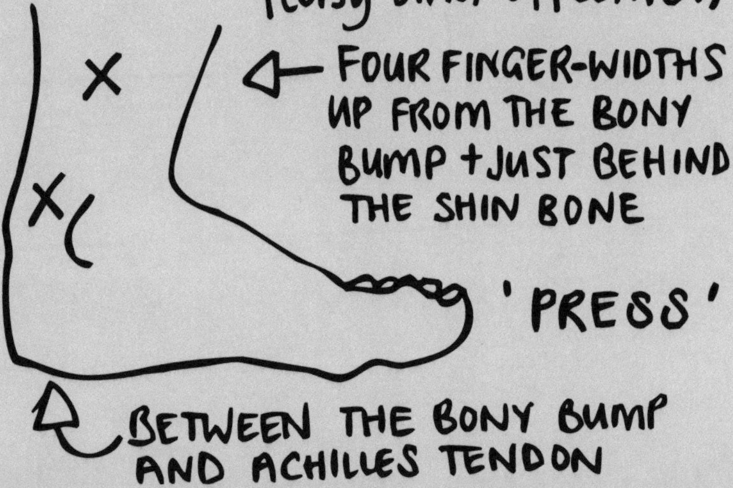

use aromatherapy oils!

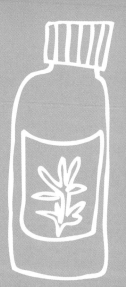

MASSAGE
LOWER BACK
USING HEEL
OF HANDS
UP AND OUTWARDS

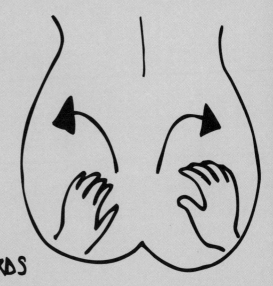

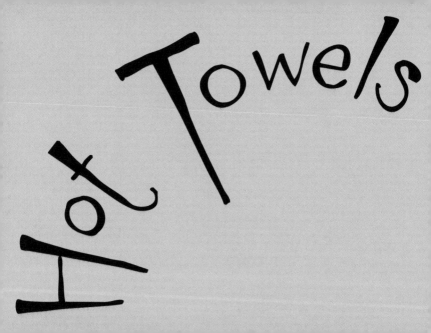

" hot water is a labouring

woman's best friend "

Dr Jennifer Barham-Floreani: Well Adjusted Babies

a relaxed mouth and throat means a relaxed perineum and cervix

make
sure
I'm not
clenching
my
teeth!

'Moo' like a cow!

Low pitched moaning and orgasmic sighs help with dilation

'Horse Lips'
-blow raspberries!

... and a
relaxed perineum is less likely to tear!

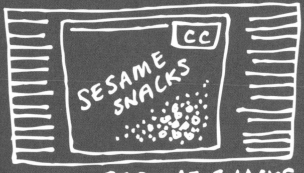

EAT SESAME SNACKS
Calcium Carbonate helps
to ease sensations of pain...

(it's true that!)

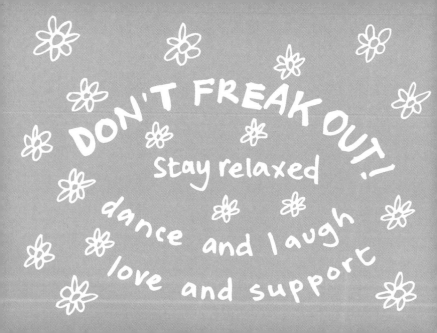

"a good belly laugh is
One of the most effective
forms of anesthesia"

Ina May Gaskin: Ina May's Guide to Childbirth

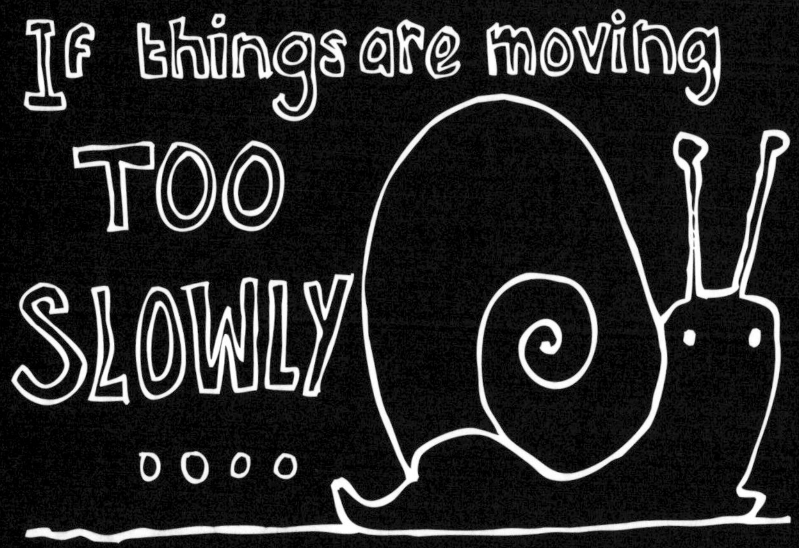
If things are moving
TOO
SLOWLY
....

Let's avoid induction

REMEMBER
HUGS
BEFORE
DRUGS

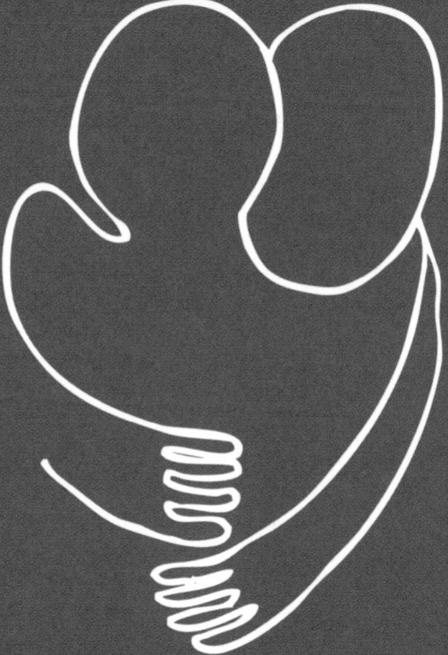

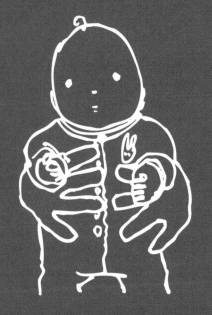

Find a new
baby to hold—
apparently
it'll send
my hormones
CRAZY!

WE CAN GO FOR A WALK AND KEEP ACTIVE OR IF WE'RE AT HOME WE CAN COOK A CURRY OR GO FOR A BUMPY RIDE IN THE CAR OR MAKE LOVE BECAUSE THIS SETS IT OFF ... OR . ....

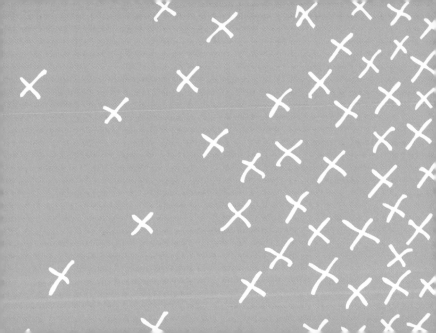

Nipple Stimulation can increase Oxytocin.

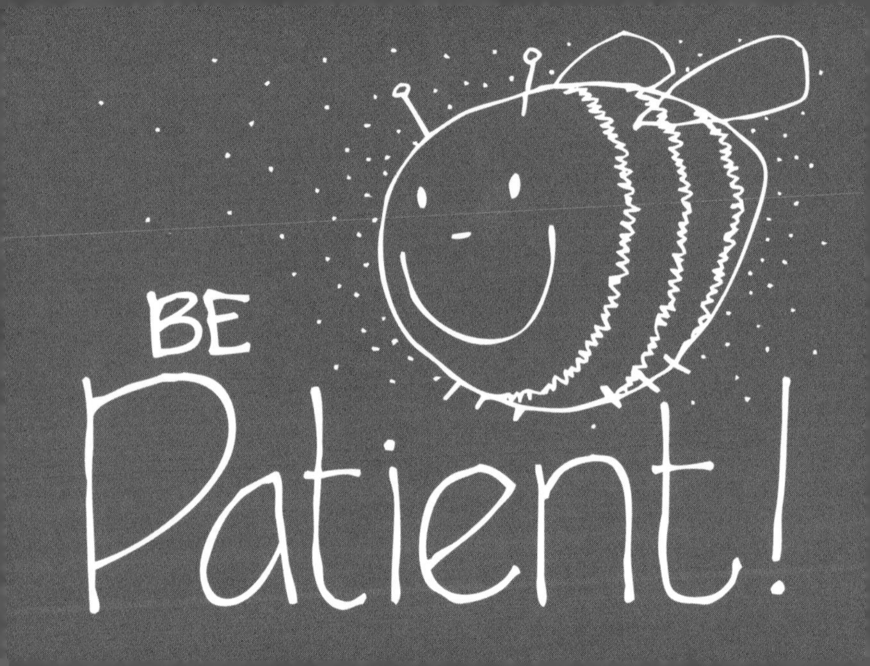
BE
Patient!

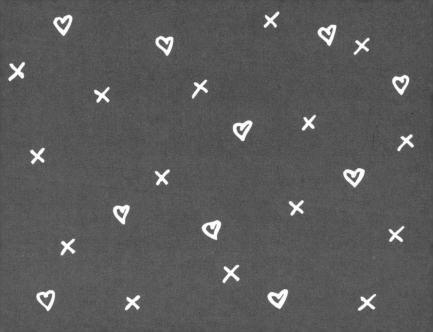

MAKE SURE THERE'S NO ADRENALIN GOING ROUND MY BODY- is there anything I'm worried about?

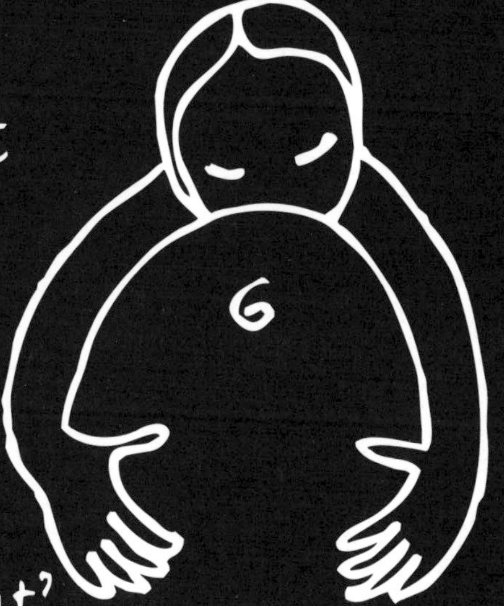

...mostly...

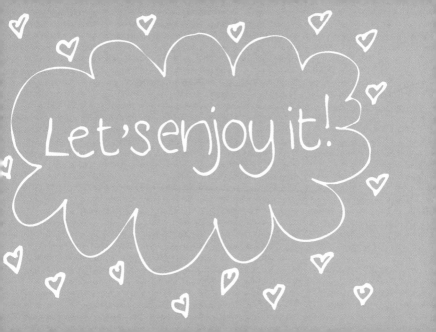

let's be excited... it's a time to celebrate!

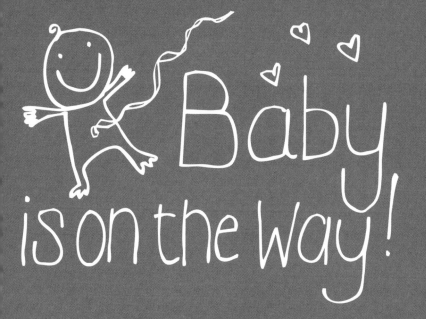

WILL BABY BE A
GIRL?

CLAIRE
TABETHA
Deisy
Jane
Bethany
SARA
KATHERYN
Mary
Rose
Jozi
ELIZABETH
Meredith
JILLY
Thea
BETH
Ellie
Kachel
Holly

FAVOURITE BABY GIRL NAMES

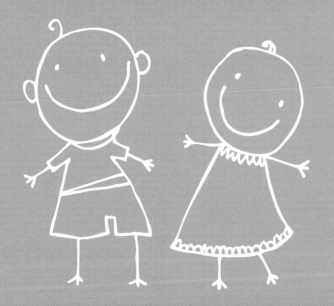

OR WILL BABY BE A

BOY?

FAVOURITE BABY BOY NAMES

James
JOE
Jonny
Adam
William
KIT
mark
Richard
HENRY
ANTHONY
Thomas
Martin
Will
FREDERICK
BILLY

I'M JUST REALLY LOOKING FORWARD TO MEETING OUR BABY!

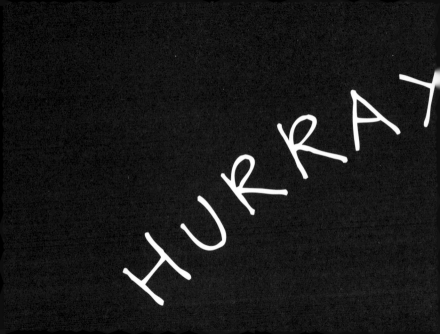

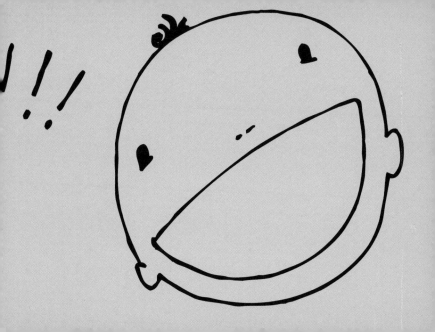

And starting

a
WHOLE
NEW
THING!

X

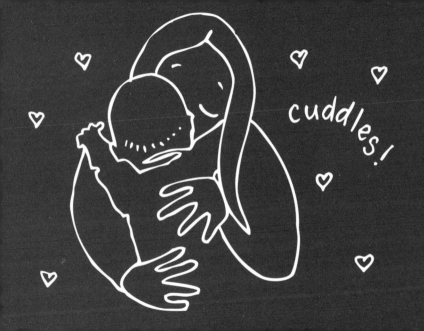

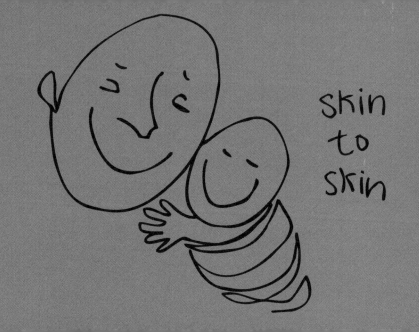

skin
to
skin

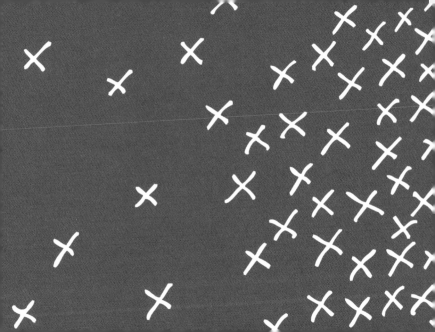

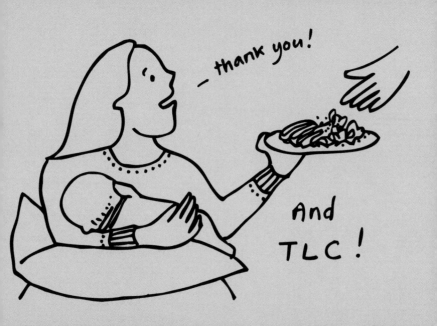

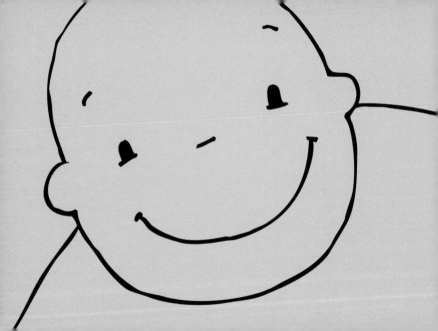

...but that's another story

TO BE CONTINUED....

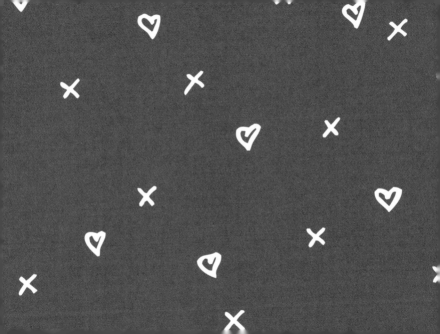

PHONE
NUMBERS

PHONE NUMBERS: FAMILY + FRIENDS